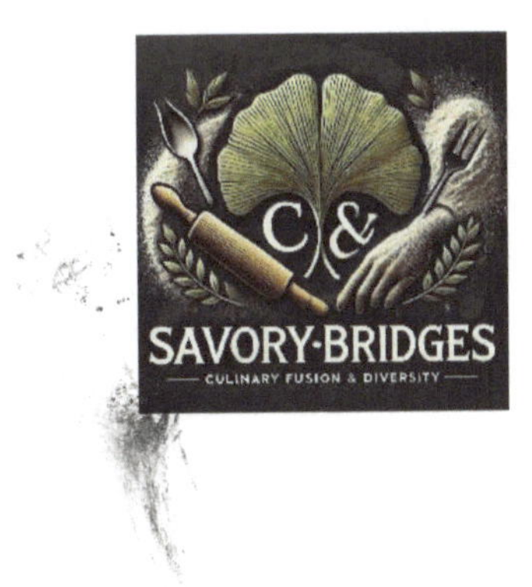

My Vegan World

The Best Healthy

Christmas Recipes

A Vegan Christmas Full of Heart, Soul, and Flavor
Close your eyes for a moment and picture a festive holiday table adorned with dishes that not only warm the heart but also speak of love—for the planet, for animals, and for yourself. Imagine the laughter of friends and family ringing through the air, the clinking of glasses in celebration, and the cozy, irresistible aroma of cinnamon, citrus, and spices filling your home. This isn't just a dream—it's your vegan Christmas, an experience that goes beyond food, offering an authentic embrace of the best this season has to offer.

"My Vegan World: The Best 10 Healthy Christmas Recipes" is more than just a recipe book—it's an invitation to step into the magic of Christmas through a lens of health, mindfulness, and creativity. It's a guide for those who want to create a Christmas that's not only a festive occasion but also a celebration of profound values: sustainability, compassion, and the joy of living in harmony with the world around us.

A Christmas That Nurtures Both Heart and Soul
Christmas is the time of year when we want to give the very best of ourselves to the people we love and the causes we believe in. But too often, this beautiful holiday is overshadowed by overindulgence, leaving us feeling weighed down—both physically and emotionally.

Choosing a vegan Christmas transforms this tradition into something even more special: a moment of **care and attention**, for our well-being and the planet's. Every ingredient you select with intention becomes a message. Every dish you prepare with love is a gift—not just for those at your table but for the Earth and future generations.

Why choose a vegan Christmas?

- **For your body:** The holidays don't have to mean guilt or excess. With dishes rich in nutrients and free from heavy, saturated fats, you can savor every bite knowing you're nourishing your body.

- **For the planet:** A vegan Christmas is a tangible act of kindness for the environment. It's a way to gift the world a celebration that treads lightly on the Earth without sacrificing the magic.
- **For the animals:** Christmas is about compassion and love. And you can honor those emotions without causing harm to other living beings.

This isn't about giving up—it's about discovering. It's not about limiting yourself—it's about expanding your horizons. This book will guide you in creating a culinary experience that will touch the hearts of everyone who gathers around your table.

What Awaits You in This Book

"My Vegan World: The Best 10 Healthy Christmas Recipes" is designed to take you on a step-by-step journey into a culinary world filled with authentic flavors, captivating aromas, and stunning presentations. Every recipe has been carefully curated to bring you the very best: dishes that blend taste, health, and simplicity.

Here's what you'll find within these pages:

- **Enchanting appetizers:** From elegant tartlets to warm and comforting soups, discover creative ways to welcome your guests with dishes that radiate elegance and warmth.
- **Showstopping main courses:** Recipes designed to take center stage, like lentil roast with pomegranate glaze or a vegan lasagna that defies all expectations.
- **Festive side dishes:** From the sweet warmth of roasted sweet potatoes to the fresh brightness of balsamic-glazed Brussels sprouts, every side dish adds a touch of magic to the table.
- **Desserts that tell a story:** Let yourself be enchanted by sweet treats that celebrate the spirit of Christmas in every bite, like spiced cookies and a vegan cheesecake that will win over even the skeptics.

A Vegan Christmas: Tradition Meets Innovation
Some may wonder if a vegan Christmas can truly feel
"complete" without the traditional staples. The answer is an
enthusiastic yes! Vegan cuisine not only respects the beloved
flavors of the season but also elevates them, offering
combinations that will surprise and delight both you and your
guests.
Every recipe in this book is designed to be:

- **Easy to prepare:** Whether you're a seasoned cook or a
  beginner, you'll find clear instructions and helpful tips
  for every recipe.
- **Balanced and healthy:** Each dish is packed with
  natural, nutrient-rich ingredients, keeping you energized
  and feeling light throughout the holidays.
- **Adaptable for everyone:** Whether your guests are
  vegan, omnivores, or have specific dietary needs, you'll
  find versatile options to please every palate.

An Invitation to Create an Unforgettable Christma
This book is not just a practical guide for your recipes, but
an invitation to reflect on what Christmas truly means. It's
a chance to open your heart to new possibilities, to
transform your kitchen into a place of creativity and joy,
and to embrace a tradition that looks toward the future.
Your '"**Vegan World**" starts here, with 10 recipes that are
not just dishes, but moments of connection, love, and
mindfulness. Are you ready to rediscover Christmas and
make it really special? Take your curiosity by the hand,
turn on the oven and get ready for a unique experience.
Welcome to a Christmas that will make your heart sing -
yours and those you love

Chapter 1: Perfect Appetizers for a Magical Vegan Christmas
In this chapter, we set the tone for a memorable vegan feast with appetizers that combine elegance, creativity, and unforgettable flavors. Designed to delight your guests from the first bite, these recipes showcase the magic of plant-based ingredients, blending creamy textures, aromatic spices, and heartwarming goodness. Whether you're hosting an intimate gathering or a grand celebration, these dishes will make the perfect introduction to your festive meal.

Recipe 1: Rustic Lentil and Mushroom Pâté Tartines
Ingredients
For the Pâté:
- 1 cup (200 g) cooked green or brown lentils
- 1 cup (150 g) cremini mushrooms, finely chopped
- 1 small onion, finely diced
- 2 cloves garlic, minced
- 2 tbsp olive oil
- 2 tbsp soy sauce or tamari
- 1 tsp thyme (fresh or dried)
- 1 tsp smoked paprika
- 2 tbsp walnuts, toasted
- 1 tbsp lemon juice
- Salt and black pepper to taste

For the Tartines:
- 6-8 slices of crusty bread, lightly toasted
- Fresh herbs (parsley or thyme) for garnish

Preparation
1. **Sauté the vegetables:**
   - Heat olive oil in a skillet over medium heat. Add the onions and cook for 3-4 minutes until translucent.

- o   Add garlic and mushrooms, cooking for another 5-7 minutes until the mushrooms release their moisture and become golden.
  - o   Stir in soy sauce, thyme, and smoked paprika. Remove from heat and let cool slightly.
2. **Blend the pâté:**
   - o   In a food processor, combine the cooked lentils, mushroom mixture, toasted walnuts, lemon juice, salt, and pepper.
   - o   Pulse until smooth but still slightly textured. Adjust seasoning if needed.
3. **Assemble the tartines:**
   - o   Spread a generous amount of the pâté onto each slice of toasted bread.
   - o   Garnish with fresh herbs and serve immediately.

Cooking Time

- Preparation: 10 minutes
- Cooking: 15 minutes
- Total: 25 minutes

Practical Tips

- Make the pâté a day ahead for enhanced flavor. Store in an airtight container in the fridge for up to 3 days.
- Use gluten-free bread for a gluten-free version.
- For added elegance, serve with a drizzle of balsamic glaze.

Nutritional Information *(Per Tartine)*

- Calories: 180
- Protein: 6 g
- Carbohydrates: 20 g
- Fat: 8 g
- Fiber: 4 g

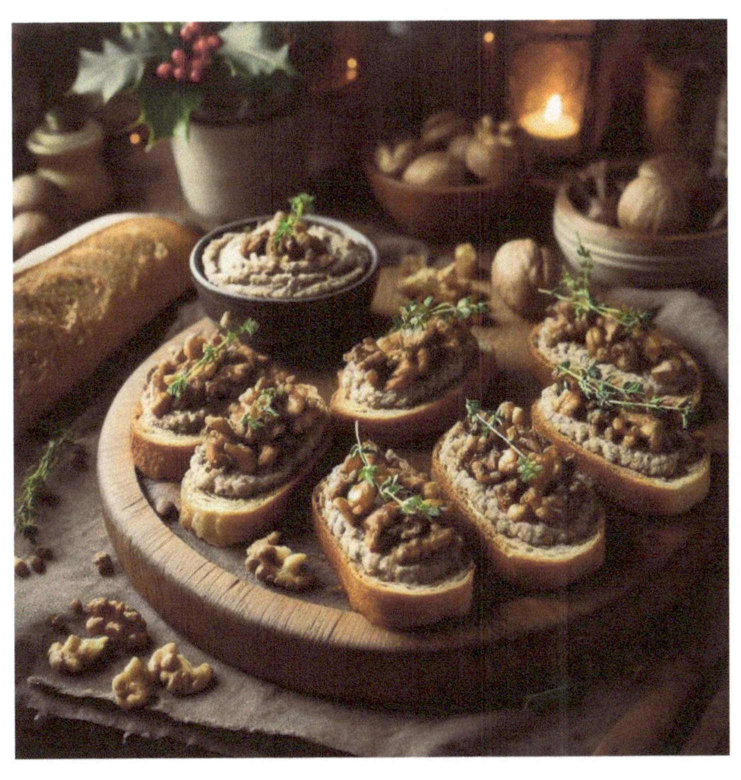

Recipe 2: Warm Pumpkin and Chestnut Soup with Spiced Croutons
Ingredients
For the Soup:

- 2 cups (400 g) pumpkin or butternut squash, peeled and diced
- 1 cup (150 g) cooked chestnuts (pre-packaged or fresh)
- 1 medium onion, diced
- 2 cloves garlic, minced
- 2 tbsp olive oil
- 3 cups (750 ml) vegetable broth
- 1/2 tsp nutmeg
- 1/2 tsp cinnamon
- 1/4 tsp cayenne pepper (optional)
- Salt and black pepper to taste
- 1/2 cup (120 ml) coconut milk

For the Spiced Croutons:

- 2 cups (150 g) cubed bread (stale bread works best)
- 2 tbsp olive oil
- 1/2 tsp smoked paprika
- 1/2 tsp garlic powder
- Salt to taste

Preparation

1. **Make the Soup:**
   - Heat olive oil in a large pot over medium heat. Add the onion and sauté for 5 minutes until softened.
   - Add garlic, pumpkin, and chestnuts, cooking for another 5 minutes.
   - Pour in vegetable broth and bring to a boil. Reduce heat, cover, and simmer for 20-25 minutes until the pumpkin is tender.
   - Blend the soup with an immersion blender or in batches in a stand blender until smooth.

     o   Stir in coconut milk, nutmeg, cinnamon, cayenne pepper, salt, and black pepper. Simmer for another 5 minutes to combine flavors.

2. **Prepare the Croutons:**
   - Preheat the oven to 375°F (190°C).
   - Toss the bread cubes with olive oil, smoked paprika, garlic powder, and salt.
   - Spread evenly on a baking sheet and bake for 10-12 minutes, flipping halfway, until golden and crispy.

3. **Serve:**
   - Ladle the soup into bowls, top with spiced croutons, and garnish with a swirl of coconut milk or fresh herbs if desired.

Cooking Time
- Preparation: 10 minutes
- Cooking: 35 minutes
- Total: 45 minutes

Practical Tips
- Roast the pumpkin in the oven beforehand for a richer flavor.
- Use canned pumpkin for a quick shortcut.
- The croutons can be made up to 3 days ahead and stored in an airtight container.

Nutritional Information (Per Serving of Soup with Croutons)
- Calories: 250
- Protein: 5 g
- Carbohydrates: 30 g
- Fat: 12 g
- Fiber: 6 g

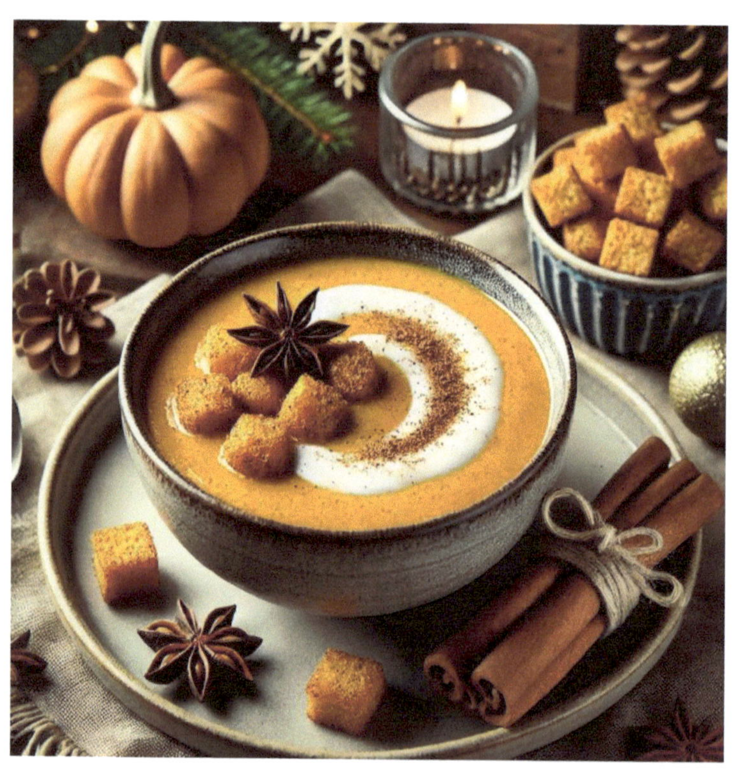

Chapter 2: Showstopping Vegan Main Courses for a Festive Celebration

The main course is the heart of every Christmas meal—a moment where the table comes alive with colors, textures, and flavors that bring joy to everyone. In this chapter, we delve into dishes designed to impress, with bold flavors and stunning presentations. Whether you're serving a cozy family dinner or hosting a grand festive feast, these recipes will become the star attractions of your vegan Christmas menu.

Recipe 1: Lentil and Walnut Roast with Pomegranate Glaze

Ingredients

For the Roast:

- 1 1/2 cups (300 g) cooked green or brown lentils
- 1 cup (100 g) walnuts, toasted and finely chopped
- 1 medium onion, finely diced
- 2 cloves garlic, minced
- 1 carrot, finely grated
- 1 celery stalk, finely chopped
- 1/2 cup (50 g) breadcrumbs (use gluten-free if needed)
- 2 tbsp ground flaxseeds + 6 tbsp water (flax egg)
- 1 tbsp soy sauce or tamari
- 1 tsp dried thyme
- 1/2 tsp smoked paprika
- Salt and black pepper to taste

For the Pomegranate Glaze:

- 1/2 cup (125 ml) pomegranate juice
- 2 tbsp maple syrup
- 1 tbsp balsamic vinegar

Preparation

1. **Prepare the flax egg:**
   - Mix the ground flaxseeds with water in a small bowl and let sit for 5 minutes to thicken.

2. **Sauté the vegetables:**
   - Heat a skillet over medium heat with a drizzle of olive oil. Sauté the onion, garlic, carrot, and celery for 5-7 minutes until softened.

3. **Mix the roast ingredients:**
   - In a large bowl, combine the lentils, walnuts, sautéed vegetables, breadcrumbs, flax egg, soy sauce, thyme, smoked paprika, salt, and pepper. Mix well.

4. **Shape and bake:**
   - Preheat the oven to 375°F (190°C). Line a loaf pan with parchment paper, press the mixture firmly into the pan, and bake for 30 minutes.

5. **Prepare the glaze:**
   - Combine the pomegranate juice, maple syrup, and balsamic vinegar in a small saucepan. Simmer over medium heat for 0 10 minutes until thickened.

6. **Glaze and serve:**

   o   After 30 minutes, remove the roast from the oven, brush with the glaze, and bake for an additional 10-15 minutes. Let rest for 5 minutes before slicing.

Cooking Time

- Preparation: 15 minutes
- Cooking: 45 minutes
- Total: 60 minutes

Practical Tips

- Make the glaze ahead of time to save prep time on the day of serving.
- Use a food processor to chop the vegetables for quicker prep.
- Leftovers make a great sandwich filling the next day!

Nutritional Information (*Per Slice*)

- Calories: 250
- Protein: 8 g
- Carbohydrates: 20 g
- Fat: 15 g
- Fiber: 6 g

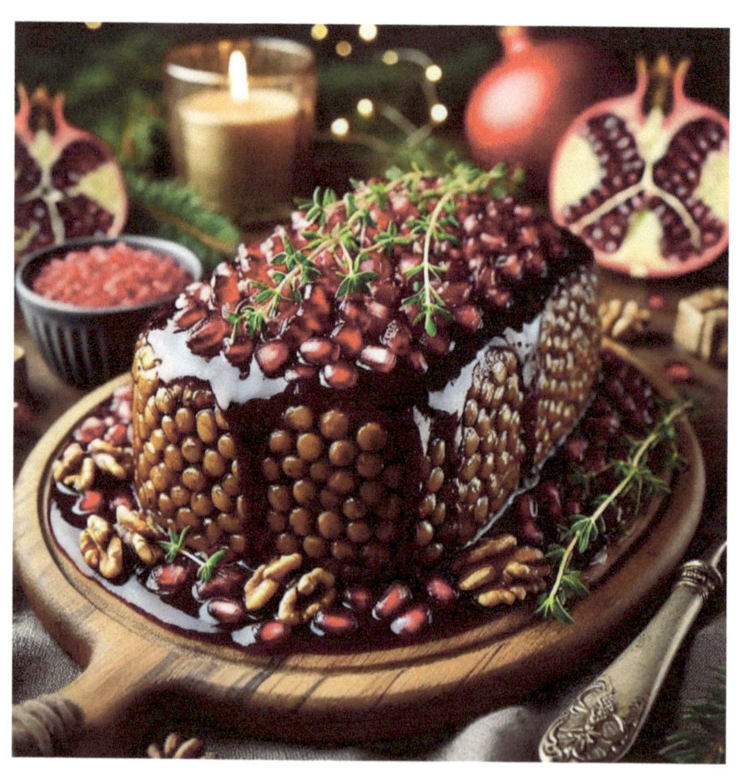

Recipe 2: Vegan Lasagna with Vegetable Ragù and Cauliflower Bechamel

Ingredients

For the Ragù:

- 1 cup (100 g) textured vegetable protein (TVP) or lentils
- 1 medium onion, finely chopped
- 2 cloves garlic, minced
- 1 carrot, finely grated
- 1 zucchini, finely diced
- 2 cups (500 ml) tomato passata
- 1 tbsp olive oil
- 1 tsp dried basil
- 1 tsp dried oregano
- Salt and pepper to taste

For the Cauliflower Bechamel:

- 2 cups (250 g) cauliflower florets
- 1 cup (250 ml) unsweetened plant-based milk
- 2 tbsp nutritional yeast
- 1 tbsp olive oil
- Salt and nutmeg to taste

For Assembly:

- 9-12 lasagna sheets (use gluten-free if needed)

- Fresh basil for garnish

Preparation

1. **Prepare the ragù:**

   - Rehydrate the TVP or cook the lentils according to package instructions.

   - Heat olive oil in a skillet over medium heat, then sauté the onion, garlic, carrot, and zucchini for 5 minutes.

   - Add the passata, basil, oregano, salt, and pepper, and simmer for 15 minutes.

2. **Make the cauliflower bechamel:**

   - Steam the cauliflower florets until tender, then blend with plant-based milk, nutritional yeast, olive oil, salt, and a pinch of nutmeg until smooth.

3. **Assemble the lasagna:**

   - Preheat the oven to 375°F (190°C). In a baking dish, layer the ragù, lasagna sheets, and cauliflower bechamel, repeating until all ingredients are used, finishing with bechamel on top.

4. **Bake:**

   - Cover the dish with foil and bake for 30 minutes. Remove the foil and bake for an additional 10-15 minutes until golden.

Cooking Time

- Preparation: 20 minutes

- Cooking: 45 minutes

- Total: 65 minutes

Practical Tips

- Let the lasagna rest for 10 minutes before slicing for cleaner servings.

- Use pre-cooked lasagna sheets to save time.

Nutritional Information *(Per Serving)*

- Calories: 300

- Protein: 10 g

- Carbohydrates: 40 g

- Fat: 8 g

- Fiber: 5 g

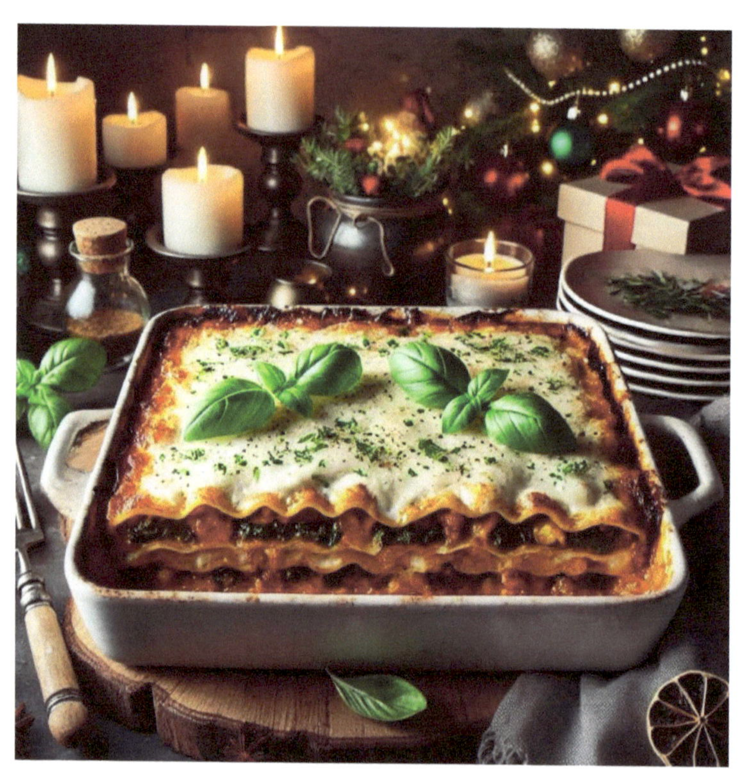

Recipe 3: Creamy Radicchio and Orange Risotto
Ingredients

- 1 1/2 cups (300 g) arborio rice
- 1 medium radicchio, finely shredded
- 1 small onion, finely chopped
- 2 cloves garlic, minced
- 1/2 cup (125 ml) white wine (optional)
- 4 cups (1 liter) vegetable broth, warmed
- Zest and juice of 1 orange
- 1 tbsp olive oil
- 2 tbsp vegan butter
- 2 tbsp nutritional yeast
- Salt and black pepper to taste

Preparation

1. **Sauté the base:**
   - Heat olive oil in a large skillet over medium heat. Sauté the onion and garlic until softened, about 3 minutes.
2. **Cook the rice:**
   - Add the rice to the skillet, stirring to coat in the oil. Cook for 1-2 minutes, then deglaze with white wine (if using).
3. **Add the liquid:**
   - Gradually ladle in the warm broth, one scoop at a time, stirring frequently and allowing the liquid to absorb before adding more.
4. **Add the radicchio and orange:**
   - When the rice is halfway cooked, stir in the shredded radicchio, orange zest, and juice. Continue cooking until the rice is creamy and tender.
5. **Finish:**
   - Stir in vegan butter, nutritional yeast, salt, and pepper. Serve hot.

Cooking Time

- Preparation: 10 minutes
- Cooking: 25 minutes
- Total: 35 minutes

Practical Tips

- Keep the broth warm to maintain the risotto's cooking temperature.
- Add more orange zest for a stronger citrus flavor.

Nutritional Information *(Per Serving)*

- Calories: 280
- Protein: 6 g
- Carbohydrates: 45 g
- Fat: 8 g
- Fiber: 4 g

Each dish embodies the warmth and creativity of a vegan Christmas feast.

Enjoy preparing these delightful main courses!

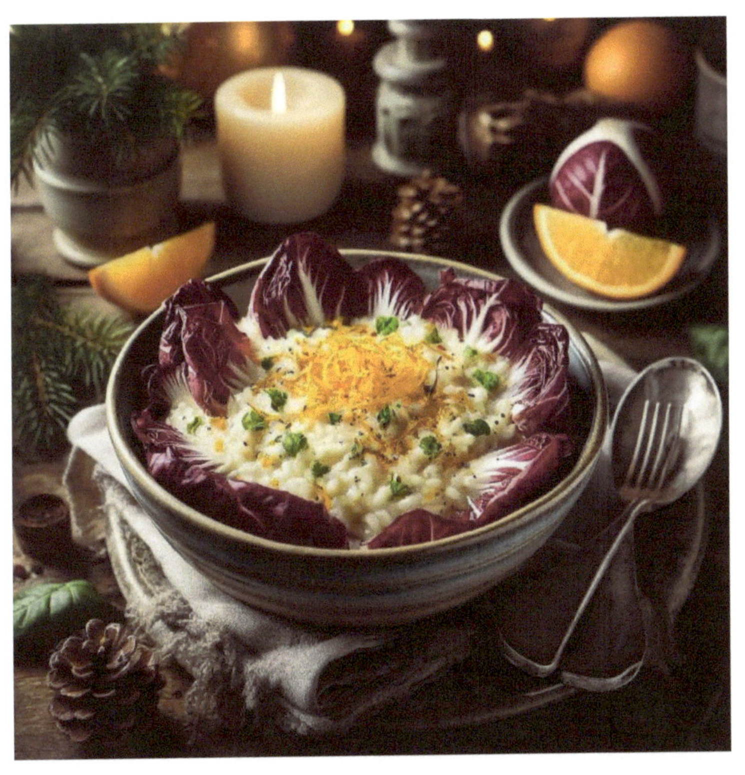

Chapter 3: Festive Side Dishes to Brighten Your Holiday Table

Side dishes are the unsung heroes of any Christmas feast, adding vibrant colors, complementary textures, and a burst of flavor to the main courses. In this chapter, we showcase two recipes that are as beautiful as they are delicious. From the crispy sweetness of roasted Brussels sprouts with almonds and cranberries to the earthy richness of sweet potatoes drizzled with tahini and lemon, these side dishes will steal the spotlight on your holiday table.

Recipe 1: Roasted Brussels Sprouts with Almonds and Cranberries

Ingredients

- 1 lb (450 g) Brussels sprouts, trimmed and halved

- 2 tbsp olive oil

- 1/2 tsp salt

- 1/4 tsp black pepper

- 1/4 cup (30 g) slivered almonds

- 1/4 cup (30 g) dried cranberries

- 1 tbsp maple syrup (optional)

Preparation

1. **Prepare the sprouts:**

   - Preheat the oven to 400°F (200°C). Toss the Brussels sprouts with olive oil, salt, and pepper in a large mixing bowl.

2. **Roast:**

   o   Spread the Brussels sprouts in an even layer on a baking sheet. Roast for 20 minutes, stirring halfway through to ensure even cooking.

3. **Add almonds and cranberries:**

   o   After 20 minutes, sprinkle the almonds and cranberries over the sprouts. Drizzle with maple syrup if using. Roast for an additional 5-10 minutes until the almonds are toasted and the sprouts are golden.

4. **Serve:**

   o   Transfer to a serving platter and enjoy warm.

Cooking Time

- Preparation: 10 minutes
- Cooking: 25-30 minutes
- Total: 35-40 minutes

Practical Tips

- For extra caramelization, add a splash of balsamic vinegar before roasting.
- Substitute pecans or walnuts for the almonds for variety.
- Use fresh cranberries for a tangier flavor, but roast them separately to prevent bursting.

Nutritional Information *(Per Serving)*

- Calories: 140

- Protein: 3 g

- Carbohydrates: 12 g

- Fat: 10 g

- Fiber: 4 g

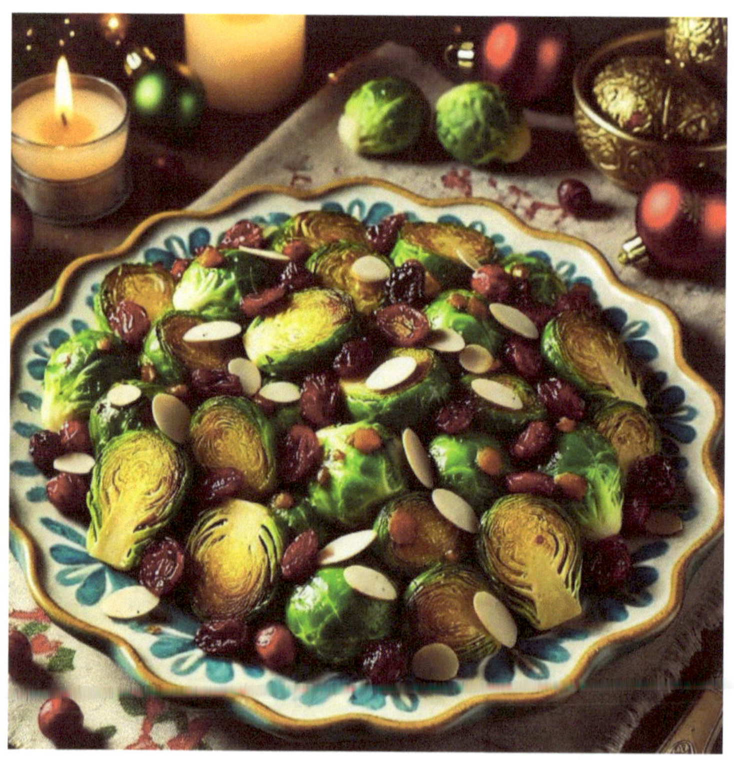

Recipe 2: Roasted Sweet Potatoes with Tahini Lemon Sauce

Ingredients

For the Sweet Potatoes:

- 2 large sweet potatoes, peeled and diced
- 2 tbsp olive oil
- 1/2 tsp smoked paprika
- 1/4 tsp garlic powder
- Salt and pepper to taste

For the Tahini Lemon Sauce:

- 3 tbsp tahini
- 1 tbsp lemon juice
- 1 tbsp maple syrup
- 2-3 tbsp water (to thin sauce)
- Pinch of salt

For Garnish:

- Fresh parsley, chopped
- Sesame seeds

Preparation

1. **Prepare the sweet potatoes:**
   - Preheat the oven to 425°F (220°C). Toss the diced sweet potatoes with olive oil, smoked

paprika, garlic powder, salt, and pepper in a
mixing bowl.

2. **Roast:**

   ○ Spread the sweet potatoes on a baking sheet in
   a single layer. Roast for 25-30 minutes, flipping
   halfway through, until tender and caramelized.

3. **Make the sauce:**

   ○ In a small bowl, whisk together tahini, lemon
   juice, maple syrup, and a pinch of salt.
   Gradually add water until the sauce reaches a
   pourable consistency.

4. **Assemble and serve:**

   ○ Arrange the roasted sweet potatoes on a
   serving plate, drizzle with tahini lemon sauce,
   and garnish with parsley and sesame seeds.

Cooking Time

- Preparation: 10 minutes

- Cooking: 25-30 minutes

- Total: 35-40 minutes

Practical Tips

- For added crunch, sprinkle roasted chickpeas over the
  sweet potatoes before serving.

- Adjust the lemon juice in the sauce to suit your taste—
  more for tartness, less for a milder flavor.

- Leftover sauce works wonderfully as a salad dressing or dip.

Nutritional Information *(Per Serving)*

- Calories: 200

- Protein: 3 g

- Carbohydrates: 25 g

- Fat: 10 g

- Fiber: 4 g

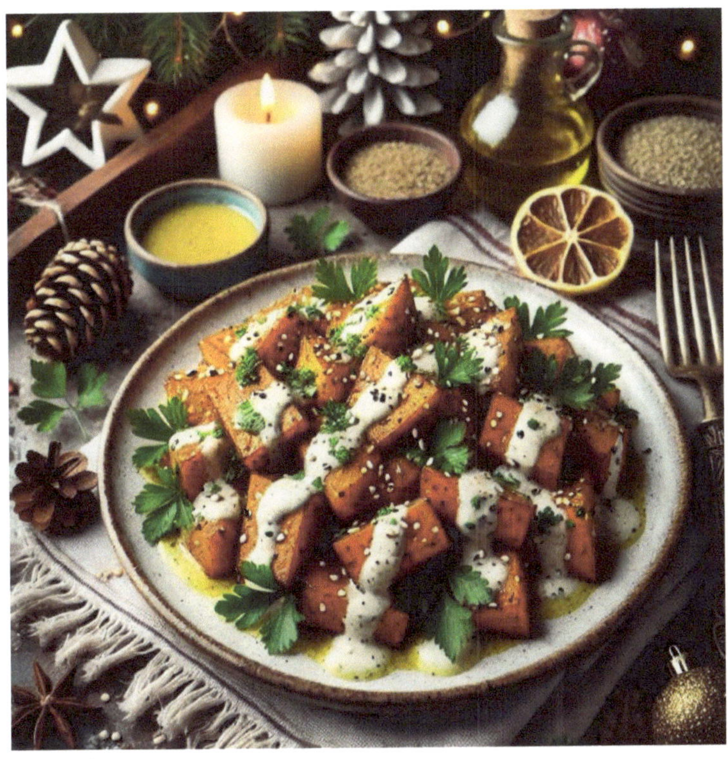

Chapter 4: Decadent Vegan Desserts to Sweeten Your Christmas

No Christmas celebration is complete without desserts, and this chapter delivers indulgent yet wholesome treats that embody the festive spirit. From spiced cookies bursting with seasonal flavors to a rich and creamy chocolate hazelnut cheesecake, and a refreshing coconut chia pudding topped with vibrant berries, these recipes will end your meal on a high note. Perfect for sharing or gifting, these desserts bring joy to every bite.

Recipe 1: Spiced Cinnamon and Ginger Cookies

Ingredients

- 2 cups (250 g) all-purpose flour (or gluten-free flour blend)
- 1/2 tsp baking soda
- 1 tsp ground cinnamon
- 1/2 tsp ground ginger
- 1/4 tsp ground nutmeg
- 1/4 tsp salt
- 1/2 cup (120 ml) coconut oil or vegan butter, softened
- 3/4 cup (150 g) brown sugar or coconut sugar
- 1/4 cup (60 ml) molasses
- 2 tbsp unsweetened plant-based milk
- 1 tsp vanilla extract

Preparation

1. **Mix the dry ingredients:**

   o   In a large bowl, whisk together the flour, baking soda, cinnamon, ginger, nutmeg, and salt.

2. **Cream the wet ingredients:**

   o   In another bowl, beat the coconut oil and sugar until smooth. Add molasses, plant-based milk, and vanilla, mixing until well combined.

3. **Combine and chill:**

   o   Gradually add the dry ingredients to the wet mixture, stirring until a dough forms. Wrap in plastic wrap and chill in the refrigerator for at least 1 hour.

4. **Shape and bake:**

   o   Preheat the oven to 350°F (175°C). Roll the dough into small balls, place them on a baking sheet lined with parchment paper, and press gently to flatten. Bake for 8-10 minutes until the edges are set. Cool completely before serving.

Cooking Time

- Preparation: 15 minutes

- Chilling: 1 hour

- Baking: 10 minutes

- Total: 1 hour 25 minutes

Practical Tips

- Sprinkle extra sugar on top of the cookies before baking for added sparkle.

- Store in an airtight container for up to a week or freeze for longer shelf life.

Nutritional Information *(Per Cookie)*

- Calories: 90

- Protein: 1 g

- Carbohydrates: 13 g

- Fat: 4 g

- Fiber: 1 g

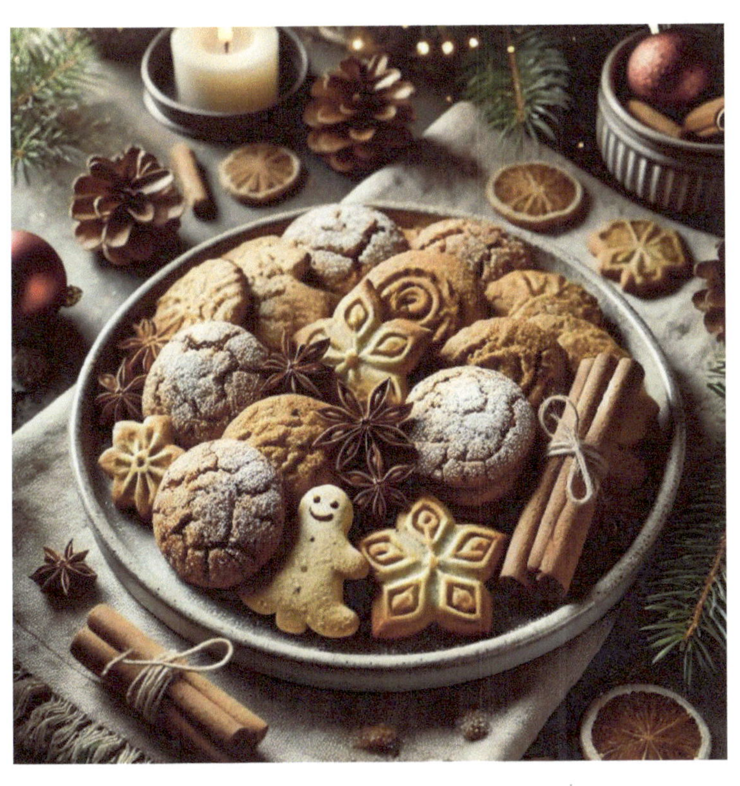

Recipe 2: Vegan Chocolate Hazelnut Cheesecake
Ingredients
For the Crust:
- 1 cup (100 g) crushed vegan biscuits or graham crackers
- 1/2 cup (50 g) hazelnuts, toasted and ground
- 1/4 cup (60 g) melted coconut oil

For the Filling:
- 2 cups (300 g) cashews, soaked overnight and drained
- 1 cup (250 ml) coconut cream
- 1/2 cup (120 g) dark chocolate, melted
- 1/4 cup (60 ml) maple syrup
- 1 tsp vanilla extract
- 1/4 cup (60 g) hazelnut butter

For Garnish:
- Dark chocolate shavings
- Crushed hazelnuts

Preparation
1. **Make the crust:**
   - Mix crushed biscuits, ground hazelnuts, and melted coconut oil. Press the mixture into the base of a springform pan and chill for 15 minutes.
2. **Prepare the filling:**
   - Blend soaked cashews, coconut cream, melted chocolate, maple syrup, vanilla extract, and hazelnut butter until smooth and creamy.
3. **Assemble and chill:**
   - Pour the filling over the crust and smooth the top with a spatula. Refrigerate for at least 4 hours, or until firm.
4. **Garnish and serve:**
   - Before serving, sprinkle with dark chocolate shavings and crushed hazelnuts.

Cooking Time

- Preparation: 20 minutes
- Chilling: 4 hours
- Total: 4 hours 20 minutes

Practical Tips

- For quicker prep, use a high-speed blender to achieve a creamy filling.
- Add a pinch of sea salt to the crust for an extra flavor dimension.

Nutritional Information *(Per Slice)*

- Calories: 300
- Protein: 5 g
- Carbohydrates: 20 g
- Fat: 24 g
- Fiber: 3 g

Enjoy these sweet treats for your vegan Christmas feast!

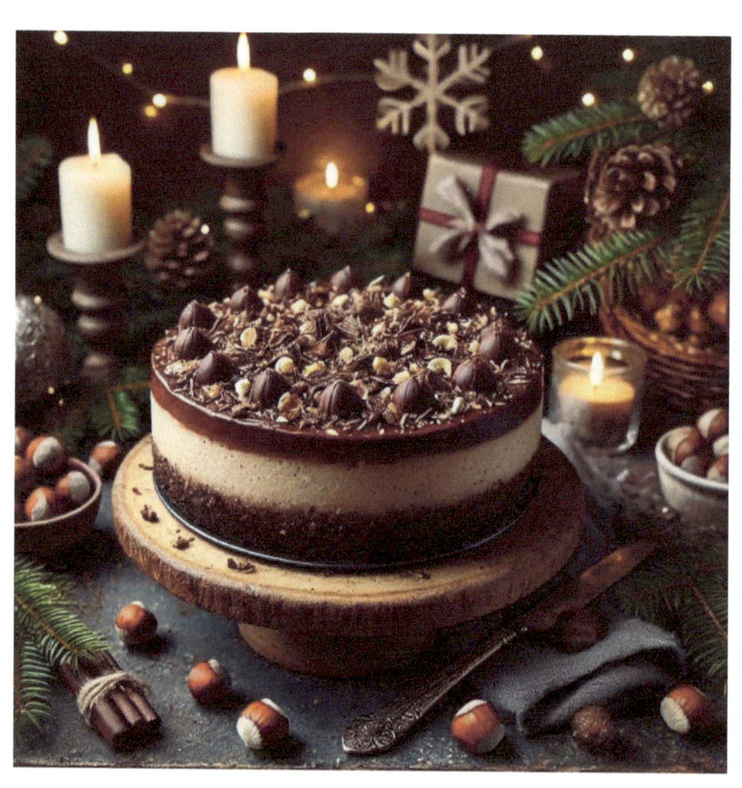

Recipe 3: Coconut Chia Pudding with Mixed Berries
Ingredients
- 1/4 cup (50 g) chia seeds
- 1 cup (250 ml) coconut milk (light or full-fat)
- 2 tbsp maple syrup or agave nectar
- 1/2 tsp vanilla extract
- 1 cup (150 g) mixed fresh or frozen berries
- 1 tbsp shredded coconut (optional, for garnish)

Preparation
1. **Mix the pudding base:**
   - In a bowl, whisk together chia seeds, coconut milk, maple syrup, and vanilla extract. Cover and refrigerate for at least 2 hours, or overnight.
2. **Prepare the berries:**
   - If using frozen berries, thaw them at room temperature. Lightly mash half of the berries to create a compote-like texture.
3. **Assemble and serve:**
   - Layer the chia pudding and berries in serving glasses or bowls. Top with additional berries and shredded coconut.

Cooking Time
- Preparation: 5 minutes
- Chilling: 2 hours
- Total: 2 hours 5 minutes

Practical Tips
- Use almond or oat milk instead of coconut milk for a lighter version.
- Add granola or nuts for extra texture and crunch.

Nutritional Information *(Per Serving)*
- Calories: 180
- Protein: 4 g

- Carbohydrates: 15 g
- Fat: 12 g
- Fiber: 6 g

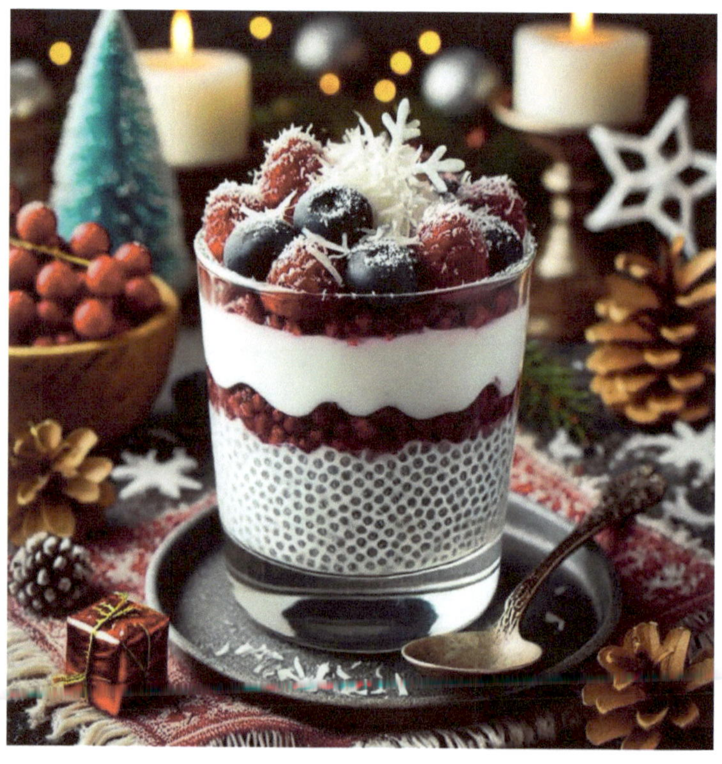

A Christmas of Flavor and Wellness

Together, we've embarked on a journey through the world of vegan Christmas, discovering recipes that not only delight the palate but also nourish the body and soul. In this eBook, *"My Vegan World: The Best Healthy Christmas Recipes"*, we've explored how a vegan diet can be incredibly diverse, flavorful, and, most importantly, healthy—even during the festive season.

Vegan Cooking and Tradition:
We've demonstrated that it's possible to enjoy cherished Christmas traditions without compromising our commitment to ethical and sustainable eating. The recipes in this book have been crafted to honor the festive spirit while adopting a more mindful approach to food.

Health and Well-being:
A central theme of this eBook is the importance of caring for our physical and mental health. The vegan recipes presented not only reduce the intake of saturated fats and cholesterol but also promote a diet rich in fiber, essential vitamins, and antioxidants.

Empathy on the Plate:
Adopting a vegan diet is more than a dietary choice—it's a way to express empathy and respect for all forms of life. During this season of giving, choosing a compassionate menu reflects the love and generosity we associate with Christmas.

An Invitation to Creativity

Vegan cooking is an open invitation to creativity. This eBook is just the beginning of your culinary journey. I encourage you to experiment, add your personal touch to these recipes, and share your creations with others. Every dish can tell a story, and every ingredient can become the start of a new Christmas tradition.

An Unforgettable Christmas

May this Christmas be an unforgettable moment of connection—not only with your loved ones but also with the world around us. Let these recipes inspire you to create a festive atmosphere that celebrates love, health, and sustainability. Remember, the true spirit of Christmas lies in giving, and what could be more precious to give than a healthier, more compassionate future for everyone?

Wishing you and your loved ones a vegan Christmas filled with joy, deliciousness, and wonder. May your tables always overflow with flavors and laughter, and may your heart be full of peace and gratitude.